# CONTENTS

# INTRODUCTION

**BASICS OF "FACE YOGA"**

If we told you that you could gain all of the face-firming, -slimming, and -tightening benefits of a facelift without ever going under the knife, would you believe it? It sounds too good to be true, but new techniques touted by skin care brands, spas, and even "gyms" for the face claim that repeating specific movements can boost circulation and lift and tighten skin over time.

TLDR: just like any other fitness regimen, exercising the muscles in your face can result in improved tone and slimness. But we're here to find out if a facial fitness routine actually be so effective as to replace plastic surgery — or even an anti-aging cream.

The health benefits, both physical and mental, of practising yoga, are manifold. But can the same apply when practising yoga with your face? Face yoga has been attributed to yield face-lifting, tightening, and sculpting benefits without salon or dermatologists' interventions. It involves working the facial muscles for improving blood circulation for a healthy glow by stimulating the production of collagen, relaxing tension on your face, de-puffing it, and also improving facial symmetry.

While we move our face every day during smiling, talking, eating, etc., facial yoga isn't simply the movement of your facial muscles. The difference is the intention with which you exercise the facial muscles to relax as well as strengthen, over time, through isolated movements.

## What Is Face Yoga?

To put it simply, face yoga is a series of facial exercises, where you intentionally isolate and tone your face muscles. We all have these tiny, delicate muscles in our face that you might not even think twice about. Take your eye area, for instance: There are over 10 muscles around our eyes constantly squinting, smiling, and expressing. "The face has muscles, just like the body," Takatsu explains. "So why not isolate and tone those muscles, relaxing the rest so you can get results?"

Of course, you move your face every day (smiling, chatting, and the like). But the kicker here is intention; like a yoga flow, you're focusing on specific muscles, strengthening them as you isolate the movement. "So many muscles are all connected; you just have to know which muscles you're using and how you want to move your muscles in a certain way."

If you think "face yoga" sounds like a fantasy, it's time to face reality: Exercising specific muscles of the face on a regular basis is not only a smart part of a healthy and mindful lifestyle, it can tone your skin and even keep annoying wrinkles at bay, some proponents say. They also believe you'll feel and look more refreshed and confident, no surgery required.

Still skeptical, or think the concept of "face yoga" sounds impossible? It's relatively easy to learn how to do yoga exercises for the face and neck. Along with eating well and getting enough sleep, these steps can make a big difference in one's appearance. Still not convinced? Even Meghan Markle has revealed she's a big fan of face yoga and swears it works, "as silly as you may feel" while doing it, as she said a few years ago in an interview.

But who cares about "silly" if you look and feel better afterward? "I knew that exercise could positively change the facial appearance because the muscles of the face work like the muscles of the body, and respond to resistance and contraction," says Annelise Hagen, founder and CEO of The Yoga Face.

Not only can exercise help the skin look healthier and more toned, Hagen says that the vast majority of us, no matter how old we are, can benefit from facial and neck revitalization stretches and movements. "Muscles respond to exercise at any age," she notes.

And with many of us on our devices for the bulk of each day, we need to know how to stretch and maintain good posture that begins, literally, at the top of our bodies. Hagen calls face yoga a "a skill set for life. And just think—it might mean you won't need injections or fillers as you age."

Be it through facial expressions or spending too much time in front of our screens, we tend to hold tension in our faces. Face yoga helps in breaking the patterns of movements through which we hold tension, like furrowing the brows, tightening the shoulders, tightening the jaw, etc. by stimulating the lymphatic system, muscles as well as the skin, relaxing it of its tension-holding patterns in the process.

The technique uses exercises and massages targeting the face, neck, and shoulders which, according to a study by the National Library of Medicine, has been found to result in a better appearance of the face due to strengthened facial muscles. Face yoga, along with reducing stress, eating well, and exercising regularly promises long-term effects in making your face look younger and tighter.

 Face yoga is a series of specific exercises for the face that are done on a regular basis. Many women report looking years younger than their biological age after incorporating the stretches and movements into their days. "It's the practice of toning the muscles of our face—and we have more than 40 of them!—to create a desired look," says Fumiko Takatsu, an internationally known anti-aging expert who created The Face Yoga Method.

Takatsu's holistic approach uses carefully developed facial exercises "that are designed to replace cosmetic procedures 100 percent naturally," she says. "By toning the muscles beneath our skin surface, we can effectively reduce wrinkles, eye bags, asymmetry issues, double chin, turkey neck, and so much more."

But is face yoga backed by science? Actually, yes, there is some evidence it can work. A study from the Northwestern University School of Medicine in 2018, for example, found that 30 minutes of daily facial exercise improved the appearance of middle-aged women across 20 weeks, giving them noticeably fuller upper and lower cheeks.

"There is some evidence that facial exercises may improve facial appearance and reduce some visible signs of aging," said lead author Dr. Murad Alam, vice chair and professor of dermatology at Northwestern University Feinberg School of Medicine when the study came out. "Assuming the findings are confirmed in a larger study, individuals have a low-cost, non-toxic way for looking younger or to augment other cosmetic or anti-aging treatments they may be seeking."

Hagen adds that we now have a body of work behind us about face yoga. "We have proof, we have documentation, and we have medical studies."

The popularity of face yoga might be due, in part, to "a backlash that is going on against a fake look" that injections, fillers, and other artificial fixes can create, she adds, especially if such measures are overused. Women want to look younger and naturally healthy without pricey upkeep or procedures.

"As we age, the skin and muscles on our face and neck naturally loosen due to our habits, loss of collagen, nutrition factors, and other aging issues," adds Takatsu. "Face yoga works by toning the muscles in our face and neck and improving blood flow and circulation. This results in healthier, glowing skin, and can help us look years younger."

She says that many women also see "results beyond the physical. Practicing face yoga encourages women to regain their confidence and embrace the aging process."

You can use face yoga techniques to target specific concerns like forehead lines, frown lines, and crow's feet. The acupressure techniques also used in face yoga can help in reducing stress, preventing headaches, releasing sinuses, and even improving the quality of your sleep. Another study by the National Library of Medicine in 2018 found that facial yoga has benefits on the mental health of elderly people as well.

every day to reap the benefits.

## How Effective Is Face Yoga?

We labor over our bodies in the gym, flexing and lifting and tensing to muscles to keep them firm and strong. Should our faces be any different? Believers in facial exercise—sometimes referred to as face yoga—believe that stimulating and building the muscles in the face can help maintain contours and elasticity, and even make us look years younger. Even cheekbone-blessed royal Meghan Markle has revealed that she does at-home (at-palace?) facial exercises to keep her face sculpted and radiant. But does it really work?

## What Is Facial Exercise?

Essentially, it's exactly what it sounds like: making repetitive motions and exaggerated expressions in order to activate and build muscles. Consider it resistance training for the face—by strengthening the matrix that holds everything up, sagging around the jaw and eyes might be less likely over time. Facial aging is caused by a loss of elasticity, as well as by the gradual displacement of fat pads between muscle and skin, which tend to slide downward over time. The idea behind doing exercises is that by building up the muscle, the fat pads will be more prone to stay in place, making the face appear fuller and more youthful.

## Does It Work?

Maybe! A 2018 study conducted at Northwestern University showed that 20 weeks of daily facial exercise did indeed yield measurably firmer skin, and fuller upper and lower cheeks. The protocol involved 30 minutes a day for the first 8 weeks of the study, then every other day thereafter. Participants—sixteen women aged between 40 and 65—deemed themselves to look up to three years younger at the study's completion, while impartial dermatologists gauged a slight but significant increase in cheek fullness. Since this was the first, and so far only, credible academic study to measure the effects of facial exercise, consider it a cautiously optimistic indication that there probably is a benefit to facial exercise—provided you dedicate a significant amount of time to it, and stick with a regimen.

"I recommend facial exercises to be done every day," says New York dermatologist Doris Day, MD. "We exercise our face every time we make expressions, and most people overuse certain muscles which ends up weakening the opposing muscles. When you frown often enough to create a crease, you're overusing those muscles and weakening the muscles that lift and smile, because you're using those muscles less. Another rule is that muscles can only pull in one direction. So for every muscle pulling down, there's an opposite/paired muscle that pulls up. I try to teach my patients (and I have a section in my book Beyond Beautiful devoted to this) how to do facial exercises to lift and rejuvenate. It helps in-office treatments last longer and in many cases it can even help delay the need for treatment."

# What Are  The Best Anti-Aging Facial Exercise To Do At Home?

The Northwestern University study involved exercises developed by Gary Sikorski of Happy Face Yoga. Two that proved to be most effective were The Cheek Lifter and the Eyebrow Lifter. For the Cheek Lifter, open the mouth to form an O, pull the upper lip up over the top teeth, and smile to lift the cheek muscles up. Then place fingers lightly on the top part of the cheek, release the muscles to lower them, and lift back up, repeating several times. For the Eyebrow Lifter, smile, then press three fingertips of each hand under your eyebrows to force your eyes open. Try to frown your eyebrows down against your fingers, then close your upper eyelids tightly and roll your eyeballs up. Hold for 20 seconds, then relax.

Day recommends what she calls The Invisible Smile: "It's all the motions of a big smile, so big that your ears move back, but without showing any teeth," she says. "This lifts the jawline, makes you feel happy and helps you be engaged and present. It's also the opposite of a frown, so you don't furrow the brows and the corners of your mouth come up."

In short, yes — but you have to be committed to the regimen. "Because facial aging is due in part to muscle loss, if you can commit to a routine, exercise may strengthen those muscles, making the entire face look more firm and youthful," explains Beauty Lab Senior Chemist Sabina Wizemann.

In one study, testers who facially exercised for 30 daily over two months, then every other day for three months, reported an increased fullness in their cheeks, making them look nearly three years younger. "It's a really great natural solution to regain your youthful appearance, and a great alternative to Botox and plastic surgery," says Koko Hayashi, facial yoga instructor at Skin Fit Gym in Los Angeles.

## What Are The Benefits?

We know yoga for the body comes with lots of benefits. But the impact of exercise on signs of facial aging hasn't been extensively studied yet. However, a 2018 study of 20 women between ages 40 and 65 showed improvements in upper and lower cheek fullness after 20 weeks of facial exercise.

Participants were also subjectively more satisfied with their outcomes than before the study.

Researchers aren't sure why this may be the case and how much it can actually help. There are theories that facial muscles could aid in keeping fat deposits in place longer, but nothing has been proven by science just yet. It also won't likely affect any existing wrinkles or sagging skin.

The verdict? A big fat maybe. But if you're on the bandwagon of keeping your face a little more taut for a little while longer, these facial exercises could be worth a try. A little self-care doesn't hurt the psyche much, either. If you can relax your face out of stress-induced brow furrows more often, all the better.

Ultimately, though, if you're aiming to look more youthful, a dermatologist or aesthetician can help you with better researched tools like a skin care routine, retinol, vitamin C, preventative Botox, and dermal fillers.

The benefits of face yoga may be more than skin deep. Touted as a natural facelift that enhances your overall well-being as well, practitioners say its benefits are immense. Research supporting these benefits is mounting.

Collins explains that face yoga promotes healthy, glowing skin.

She says: "Face yoga helps to lift and firm the muscles under the skin, which smooths lines and wrinkles. Massage helps to boost circulation, improve lymphatic drainage, and release tension. Acupressure techniques boost circulation and relieve stress, which can aid in preventing headaches, releasing sinuses, and enhancing the quality of your sleep."

Collins also says that face yoga exercises can relax overactive muscles while toning weaker muscles, which helps to prevent sagging and expression lines.

A small 2018 Trusted Source study investigated the effectiveness of 32 facial exercises in reducing the appearance of aging in middle-aged women.

For the first 8 weeks, the participants did daily 30-minute sessions of face exercises. During the next 12 weeks, they did the sessions every other day.

Most of the women showed improvements to the fullness of their faces and were highly satisfied with the visible results. They reported significant improvement in 18 of 20 facial features. Further in-depth research is required to expand upon these findings.

Another small 2018Trusted Source study examined the benefits of facial exercises in improving the mental health of older people. The participants did 30-minute facial exercise sessions twice-weekly for 12 weeks, which included yogic breathing as well as rhythmic facial movement, muscle stretching, and facial yoga. The results reported positive improvements related to mental health, facial expression, and tongue muscle power.

However, a 2014 reviewTrusted Source of the literature included nine studies about the benefits of face yoga and other facial exercises for facial rejuvenation. The researchers concluded that more research was needed and the results of all nine studies were inconclusive. They found the results were subjective since the studies were small and all relied on study authors and participants to determine the success of the interventions.

Some anecdotal reports say face yoga and massage may be effective for improving facial appearance, suggesting it enhances mindfulness and awareness as well.

As practitioners learn to strengthen or relax certain muscles, they may experience improved posture, fewer headaches, and reduced teeth grinding. Others say they find it easier to relax and fall asleep at night.

In addition to the reported reduction of the appearance of fine lines and wrinkles, face yoga may promote increased lymphatic drainage leading to reduced puffiness and improved circulation. Face yoga practitioners also report it may help to:

- control face muscles
- promote proper nostril breathing
- firm the neckline
- reprogram muscle memory
- improve symptoms of temporomandibular joint (TMJ) disordersTrusted Source
- make your face more symmetrical
- reduce the appearance of dark underage circles
- improve confidence
- tone face muscles
- correct sagging
- generate positive emotions
- make your face less rounded

Face yoga's main praise is its effects on the skin's appearance—namely, tightening the skin and keeping it plump. By stimulating the blood flow in your face, the circulation can spur the production of collagen (which as we know keeps your skin looking firm and taut) and delay the appearance of fine lines and wrinkles. One 2018 study even found that the daily exercise could reduce signs of facial aging, with improvements especially in upper and lower cheek fullness.

You might be thinking: Isn't constantly moving your face what causes those wrinkles? And you're right—we emote quite a bit throughout the day, making the face a vulnerable spot for fine lines. But by intentionally toning those facial muscles, you can promote blood circulation in the skin and actually help tighten the area. "You're not causing any unwanted wrinkles because you're controlling the movement," says Takatsu.

Even more so, the practice helps you become aware of those unconscious expressions you might not think twice about (like, say, a furrowed brow as you slouch over your desk). "I truly believe 20% of the benefits is the exercise itself, but 80% of the results come from the fact that you're paying attention to your facial expressions throughout the day," Takatsu explains. "You catch yourself tightening your shoulders or tensing the forehead."

## Other Benefits Of Face Yoga

### • Softened wrinkles and plumped skin

With age, natural collagen levels decrease. As a result, the skin starts to sag and loses tone, and wrinkles become more pronounced. The advantage of face yoga exercises is that they don't just stimulate muscles; they also stimulate the production of collagen and elastin. By practicing face yoga regularly, you'll tone up your skin, visibly reduce the depth of wrinkles, and make your face look smoother and less tired.

### • A Way To De-Stress

When you perform face yoga exercises, you'll probably find that you feel more relaxed! These exercises are good for both the body and mind, as they relax facial muscles while acting on the nervous system, reducing stress. If your skin reacts easily to stress and often shows signs of sensitivity and redness, try combining face yoga exercises with La Cure Peau Calme. This soothing treatment softens the skin, and relieves and reduces sensitivity within just 15 days. Enriched with soothing Blond Psyllium, calming Blue Daisy and protective Poria Cocos, it supports your skin's balance and provides it with long-lasting protection.

## . Gravity-Fighting Facial Exercises

There are around fifty muscles in the face, but they don't get a workout every day! This means that they may lose tone prematurely – and there is a direct correlation between this loss of tone and skin aging. You can help your face to defy gravity by practicing the following exercises every day for five minutes.

## • Smooth Forehead Lines

To soften and smooth forehead lines, begin by placing your palms on the top of your forehead. Breathe in deeply and push the skin of your forehead upward. Continue to hold the skin in this position as you breathe out and look down as far as possible. Repeat ten times.

## • Reduce Frown Lines Between The Eyes

These vertical frown lines are formed by repeated contractions of the muscles between the eyebrows. To soften them, begin by stretching the eyebrows with deep smoothing movements, starting from the middle of the face (where the frown lines are) and working outward. Repeat ten times.

Next, apply even pressure with the palm of your hand on the frown lines, while breathing in and out deeply. Repeat this exercise five times.

## • Make Your Eyes Look More Open, And Smooth Crow's-Feet

To smooth the eye area, place three fingers (index, middle and ring) on your temples, then pull your skin back, applying moderate pressure, for five seconds. For an even firmer "grip," place your thumbs below your jawbone. Repeat this exercise five times.

## • Reduce Nasolabial Folds And Firm The Cheeks

Also known as "smile lines," nasolabial folds are expression lines that go from the sides of the nose down to the corners of the lips. This exercise helps to smooth these lines while also working on the cheeks, for a firming effect. Fill your cheeks with air and hold the position for five seconds. Then transfer the air from one cheek to the other, holding it for five seconds each time. To work on smile lines, move the air to the upper mouth and puff out your upper lip, then puff out your lower lip. Repeat this exercise five times, holding each position for five seconds.

To avoid puckering the lips during this exercise (you don't want to create new wrinkles!), you can place one finger on your mouth to hold it still.

## • Plump The Lips

The lips also lose volume with age: they gradually become thinner, and their outline becomes less defined. This exercise will strengthen the muscles around the mouth and help plump the lips. Breathe in and tilt your head slightly backward, making sure the position is comfortable. Breathe out, blowing about ten exaggerated "big kisses" up into the air.

Extra benefit: this exercise is also good for the cheeks and jawline.

## • Redefine Facial Contours

A loss of firmness and definition around the jawline is one of the first signs of aging. This simple exercise provides a natural way to redefine and tone facial contours. Cup your chin in your hands so your hands are clasping your jawline, all the way up to the ears. Breathe in, then tilt your head forward so that you're exerting pressure while resisting with the hands (you could place your elbows on a table to make this movement easier). Hold the position for five seconds while breathing out. Repeat five times.

In addition to your daily face yoga exercises, don't forget to use a skincare routine that's tailored to your skin's needs. To help you choose the most suitable products, you can take our online skin diagnosis. You'll get answers in just 3 minutes!

## Is There A Cheat?

Not exactly. But there is a different approach: stimulating the facial muscles with massage. This is the theory behind the wildly successful FaceGym, founded by Inge Theron, formerly the Spa Junkie columnist for the Financial Times. "I really wanted the workout to mimic what you do in the gym," she says. So each facial involves a warm up, followed by "cardio for draining and detoxifying," then "sculpting, for the toning and tightening the muscles." She considers is "a personal training studio for the scaffolding of the face.Our trainers go through an intensive 3-week boot camp to learn and perfect the deep tissue massage and muscle manipulation techniques, which are used along with the addition of tools such as the FaceGym Pro, Face Ball, Guasha Stone and Gold Roller. It's the unique combination of muscle work, tools and highly efficacious skincare that provide dramatic results."

Celebrity facialist Thuyen Nguyen, who regularly works with Michelle Williams, Cindy Crawford, and Amal Clooney, espouses a similar concept with his FaceXercise, but he believes that all of the work can be done with the h\\ ands—no microcurrent or rollers required [which he says can deliver better results, and more quickly, than facial exercise alone could ever do]. "It's very difficult for people to keep facial exercise up, because they have to do it for 20 to 30 minutes a day. Most of us barely have time to shower," he says. "When you're 20 something years old, you don't even have to work out and your muscle tone is held because your metabolism is so fast. But five to ten years later, your body just doesn't keep the muscle tone, so you have to work out more. It's the same philosophy for skin. I just do the work while the clients lie back."

The difference, he says, between active facial exercise, which can strengthen muscles, and passive facial exercise—delivered through massage—is that the former "can't help with elasticity or with pores," while the latter can. "You see the tone come back," he says, "and just like when you work out the body, you raise your endorphins, you raise your immune system, and your skin gets a glow from all of the blood circulation." Nguyen typically sees clients once a or once a month, depending on schedule and budget. "But when I start with most people, I have them come back one week after the first session, because just like a trainer I'm capturing muscle memory. The more I push the blood in, the more cheek expands, and the more they work with me the more resilient their skin and muscles become. Just like the body looks better and feels less lethargic the more you exercise, it's the same with the face."

This content is imported from {embed-name}. You may be able to find the same content in another format, or you may be able to find more information, at their web site.

Facialist Joanna Czech believes that the best approach is a combination of regular facials involving microcurrent with an at-home regimen of muscle-stimulating massage—and if you have the time to do facial exercises, go for it. "I recommend facial massage to all my clients," she says. "It's different from facial exercise, and it's what I consider the lazy way to stimulate your muscles and skin. It can actually change the shape of your face, lifting the brow and jawline and sculpting the cheekbone. It stimulates blood flow, bringing more oxygen and nutrients to the tissue and results in a brighter, healthier complexion. All of my treatments include facial massage, but I cannot do facial exercises on clients—they have to do those themselves."

## Which Types Of Yoga Might Be Better For Your Face?

Nothing the benefits of yoga asana, traditional ways of sitting during yoga, Collins explains: "Forward folds bring fresh blood and oxygen to the skin, which promotes a healthy glow. Backbending poses tone and firm the front neck muscles, while twists firm the side of the face and release neck tension."

Slower types of yoga that involve holding poses for extended periods may give you more of an opportunity to bring this awareness to your facial muscles. This includes Hatha, Yin, or restorative yoga. You can also work on relaxing your face muscles during your mediation, pranayama, or yoga nidra practice.

Work on bringing awareness to your face during traditional yoga postures. Observe if you're holding onto any tension or making facial expressions. Notice if you're concentrating on relaxing your face so intently that you end up furrowing your brow or lifting your eyebrows.

Some teachers cue the Buddha smile or Mona Lisa smile to indicate a relaxed face with the corners of your mouth turned upward slightly.

## Which Specific Areas Can Doing Face Yoga Exercise Help?

Depending on your concerns and goals, Collins says you can use face yoga to target any area of your face. Tension tends to build in your forehead, brows, and jaw. If you have tightness in any of these areas, build your routine around these places. Wrinkles are common around the forehead, eyes, and mouth.

To reduce the appearance of wrinkles in certain areas, choose massages and exercises that target these places. Or you can choose exercises designed to alleviate specific concerns such as headache, insomnia, or sinus infection.

## How To Do Face Yoga.

Before diving into the poses, here's what you need to know:

## How Often Do You Need To Practice Face Yoga To See Results?

"Ideally every single day, if you want to see good results," says Hayashi. Wizemann agrees that consistency is the only key to success: "If you like a challenge and can stick to a 30-minute daily beauty routine for at least five months, you could possibly look a couple of years younger." But Wizemann adds that these exercises shouldn't replace the proven efficacy of anti-aging skin care and sun protection. Ideally, Takatsu says to practice face yoga twice a day. Once in the morning to wake your face muscles up and again before bed to release all the tension you've accumulated during the day. "It can be as little as five minutes."

In terms of how many poses per session, she notes four to five (for 30 seconds each) will do the job just fine. All you need is a quick warmup, then you're able to focus on specific muscles you want to target.

## How Does Face Yoga Work?

In facial fitness classes like Hayashi's (which run $200 per 50-minute session), you'll learn to "wake up your sleeping muscles in your face" to improve tone (she says 80% of them lay dormant), and "relax your facial muscles, especially your over[worked] muscles which cause wrinkles" she explains. To smooth wrinkles and firm up saggy spots, Hayashi shared her five best face yoga exercises. You might feel silly making these faces at first, but the results speak for themselves.

Don't be fooled, It's hard. You might even find yourself unintentionally holding your breath or tensing up as you hold a pose. Because those facial muscles are so small and delicate, it's difficult to isolate and activate the muscle you're trying to target. That's why, Takatsu says, beginners might want to start with toning the bigger muscles first (such as the neck and forehead area) before moving to more delicate places like the eyes. She compares the process to riding a bike—it's difficult at first, but once you get used to the movement, it feels quite natural.

# 5 Poses For Beginners.

Below, a beginner-friendly face yoga flow. As Takatsu advises, we'll start with the bigger muscles first, then dive into the more delicate areas like the eyes and mouth. Friendly heads-up: During each pose, be sure to keep your posture straight, keep your chest open, and keep breathing. (It's harder than it sounds!)

## 1.  Warm Up

KOKO HAYASHI / SKIN FIT GYM

How to do the exercise: Start your "workout circuit" by blowing exaggerated raspberries not only just with the lips, but with the cheeks as well. "The bigger vibration is better for relaxing facial muscles," says Hayashi. "Lip muscles are a core muscle for the face. By relaxing these muscles, other muscles are relaxed too."

How often to do it: At least once (and up to three times) per day, "or whenever you feel stressed," says Hayashi. Or For allover blood circulation, this is your go-to, simple pose.

Drop your jaw as if you're yawning, feeling that sensation you're creating in the cheek area.

Without moving your forehead, move your gaze from eye-level, all the way past your forehead to the ceiling without moving your forehead muscles.

Hold for 10 seconds, remembering to breathe throughout.

Repeat two times for a total of 30 seconds.

## 2. Slim Your "Tech Neck" Double Chin
KOKO HAYASHI / SKIN FIT GYM

How to do the exercise: Keeping your shoulders down and relaxed, tip your chin up to the ceiling until you feel a good stretch in the upper neck and chin area. Then, alternate making duck lips and sticking out your tongue, holding each "pose" for 5 seconds each. Repeat three times.

Make sure to keep your chin extended and keep your neck taut the whole while. Hayashi reminds that this should feel a bit strenuous: "If you don't get tired, it's not effective."

How often to do it: 1-2 times per day.

This pose releases tension and tones the neck area. The neck and jaw are connected by the platysma muscle, says Takatsu, so this stretch can also tone your jawline as well.

Relaxing the shoulders, move your chin to one side, slightly up at a 45-degree angle.

Pucker your lips into a kiss.

Hold for 10 seconds, remembering to breathe throughout.

Switch sides and repeat. Repeat both sides two times for a total of 30 seconds on each side.

## 3.  Smooth Smile Lines

KOKO HAYASHI / SKIN FIT GYM

How to do the exercise: First off, don't stop smiling and laughing! "If you don't smile, you're not going to develop cheek muscle," says Hayashi. Instead, tackle smile lines by "breaking down the tension in the muscle from the inside out by using the tongue."

Starting up by the nose, where Hayashi says the lines tend to be deepest, "stick your tongue inside your mouth and make a tiny circle on the labial line." Do five circles clockwise and counterclockwise on each side to smooth smile lines.

How often to do it: once per day

For the forehead. forehead freeze pose

Image by Fumiko Takatsu

Takatsu calls this pose the "instant pick-me-up." That's because it doubles as a meditation, she explains, as you embrace the energy of your surroundings (great for a morning face yoga ritual).

Place your fingers in a downward V-shape on the forehead, pulling up slightly.

Keeping your shoulders relaxed and chin slightly up, breathe in and out for 10 seconds.

Run the palms down the sides of the face, closing your eyes and reveling in the sensation.

Repeat two times for a total of 30 seconds

## 4.  For The Eyes.

binocular eyes pose

Image by Fumiko Takatsu

To target the delicate under-eye area, this pose isolates the lower lid movement, as well as the forehead muscles. The key here, Takatsu says, is to try not to wrinkle your forehead.

Curl your hand into a "C" shape. Place your index fingers above the eyebrow, along the upper eye bones.

Position your thumb on the side of your nose, just above the nostril. Press your fingers downward and then sideways.

Keeping your shoulders relaxed, open your eyes as wide as possible. Hold for five seconds, while pressing your index finger firmly into your eyebrow making sure your eyebrow and forehead don't move.

Squint the eye five times, before closing your eyes and relaxing for a few seconds.

Repeat two times for a total of 30 seconds. Repeat on the other side..

Firm Up Saggy Cheeks and Jowls

KOKO HAYASHI / SKIN FIT GYM

How to do the exercise: "Bulldog face is cute for dogs but not cute for us," says Hayashi. "To remove the saggy cheeks, pull everything to the side: imagine your right teeth pulled to the left side of your mouth" in what should look kind of like a sideways kissy-face. Hold for 10 seconds for an effective exercise that "trains and stretches at the same time. It is a great way to improve skin elasticity," Hayashi says.

How often to do it: 3-5 times per day, for best results

## 5.  Fight Eye Wrinkles And Crow's Feet

KOKO HAYASHI / SKIN FIT GYM

How to do the exercise: Keeping shoulders back and relaxed, point your chin down to your chest and make an oval with your mouth. At the same time, look upward with just the eyes: "don't move your head or shoulders, you should feel stretching underneath the eye," says Hayashi.

Hold for three seconds, and then tuck the upper lip inside the mouth to make an "ahh" face. This circuit should give you "a deep stretch in the face … so that wrinkles don't stay."

How often to do it: Once a day, no more. Otherwise, you risk bringing "too much stretch" to the skin and the muscles in the face.

As we know, our lips thin as we age due to a loss of collagen. This pose works to stimulate the lip barrier, for naturally full, plump lips.

Place your index fingers on the corners of your mouth.

Smile, showing the entire row of your front teeth. Make sure the corners of your mouth are at the same level.

Curl your tongue up slightly, and take 5 seconds to slowly move it to one side. Take 5 seconds to move your tongue to the other side.

Repeat two more times for a total of 30 seconds, remembering to breathe throughout.

Face yoga is actually quite similar to the other types of yoga—you're toning the muscles, getting your blood flowing, and getting some meditation and breathwork in while you're at it. And just like yoga, it may take a bit of practice before you finally get the hang of the exercise. But start with these five poses—just twice a day—and you might notice some changes in your complexion.

## 7 Yoga Exercise For Your Face

For each exercise, work to your comfort level. You may feel warmth or heat, but you shouldn't experience pain or discomfort.

Always start with clean hands and a clean face. Use an oil, serum, or cleansing balm so your fingers can glide easily over your skin without it being too slippery. Massaging oils or serums into your skin can help the product penetrate your skin for deeper absorption.

## 1. Tension Relief

Stimulating this acupressure point helps to reduce eye strain. You can use it to calm down during the day or before you fall asleep.

Press into the inner corner of your eyes for 30 seconds.

Then circle gently in one direction for 30 seconds.

Repeat in the opposite direction.

## 2. Eye Circles

This exercise boosts oxygen circulation and alleviates puffiness. Use light, featherweight touches.

Place your ring fingers at the inside of your eyebrows.

Gently tap your fingers toward the outside of your eyebrows.

Press into your temples for a few seconds.

Continue to tap above your cheekbones to the inner corner of your eyes.

Continue for 30 seconds.

## 3. Brow Smoother

This exercise relaxes the frontalis muscle, which is the large muscle at the front of your forehead. Often this muscle is over-used, which can cause stiffness, rigidity, and expressions of stress.

Place your fingertips at the center of your forehead, facing inwards.

Gently press your fingertips into your forehead as you move your fingers toward your temples.

Release your fingers.

Continue for 30 seconds.

## 4. Neck Massage

This exercise boosts lymphatic drainage and alleviates neck tension. It helps to correct sagging skin around your jaw and neck.

Tilt your head back slightly.

Place your fingers at the top of your neck.

Apply gentle pressure as you glide your fingers down to your collarbone.

Press into your collarbone for a few seconds before releasing your fingers.

Continue for 30 seconds.

## 5. Jaw Unlocker

This exercise engages the muscles in your jaw and neck.

While seated, make a fist with your left hand and place it on the outside of your jaw with your thumb facing down.

Turn your head toward your fist, feeling a stretch on the side of your neck.

Don't allow your hand to move.

Then press your jaw toward your hand for a few seconds.

Gently release.

Repeat on the opposite side.

## 6. Lion's Breath

Also known as Lion's pose, this is a yogic breathing exercise that reduces stress and relaxes your face muscles.

From a seated position, lean forward to brace your hands on your knees or the floor.

Inhale deeply through your nose.

Open your mouth wide, stick out your tongue, and stretch your tongue toward your chin.

Forcibly exhale your breath across the base of your tongue while making a "ha" sound.

Relax and breathe normally.

Repeat up to 7 times.

Breathe deeply for 1 to 3 minutes.

## 7. Face Tapping

Tapping promotes relaxation and boosts circulation.

Start at your forehead and use your fingertips to rhythmically tap your skin.

Continue all along your face toward your jaw.

Next, tap the front of your neck and across your shoulders.

Then move up along the back of your neck to your head.

Finally, rub your palms together to generate heat.

Cup your hands over your face and breathe deeply for several breaths.

# Facial Exercises: Are They Bogus?

While the human face is a thing of beauty, maintaining taut, smooth skin often becomes a source of stress as we age. If you've ever searched for a natural solution to sagging skin, you may be familiar with facial exercises.

Fitness celebrities have long endorsed facial workouts designed to slim the face and reverse the aging process — from Jack LaLanne in the 1960s to soccer star Cristiano Ronaldo in 2014. But do these exercises actually work?

Countless books, websites, and product reviews promise miraculous results, but any evidence that suggests facial exercises are effective for slimming

cheeks or reducing wrinkles is largely anecdotal.

There's little clinical research on the efficacy of facial exercises. Experts like Dr. Jeffrey Spiegel, chief of facial plastic and reconstructive surgery at Boston University School of Medicine, believe that these muscle-blasting facial workouts are a total bust.

However, a small studyTrusted Source conducted by Dr. Murad Alam, vice chair and professor of dermatology at Northwestern University Feinberg School of Medicine and a Northwestern Medicine dermatologist, shows some promise of the possibility of improvement with facial exercises. Assuming that a larger study supports the same results, it may not be time yet to give up on facial exercises.

## Why Don't They Work For Weight Loss?

Generally speaking, exercising muscles burns calories, which can mean weight loss. However, we don't decide where in the body those calories come from. So, while facial exercises may strengthen your muscles, if what you're after are slimmer cheeks, rhythmic smiling alone won't get you there.

Spiegel notes that "spot reduction," or working out a particular area of the body to lose weight there, does not work. Other experts agree. The only healthy, nonsurgical way to reduce facial fat is overall weight loss achieved through diet and exercise. In fact, working out your facial muscles can have undesirable effects, such as making you appear older.

## For Wrinkle Reduction

The muscles in the face form a complex web and can attach to bone, each other, and the skin. Unlike bone, skin is elastic and provides little resistance. As a result, working out facial muscles pulls on the skin and will stretch it out, not tighten it.

"The truth is that many of our facial wrinkles come from excess muscle activity," Spiegel says. Laugh lines, crow's feet, and forehead wrinkles all come from using facial muscles.

The idea that toning facial muscles prevents wrinkles is backward, notes Spiegel. "It's like saying 'stop drinking water if you're thirsty,'" he says. "The opposite works." Botox, for example, prevents wrinkles by freezing muscles, which eventually atrophy. Patients with partial facial paralysis often have smoother, less-wrinkled skin where they're paralyzed.

## What Does Work?

The primary nonsurgical way to slim down in your face is to slim down as a whole, with diet and exercise. Everybody is different, though, and a fuller face may be the result of bone structure, rather than fat.

If preventing wrinkles is your goal, simple steps like using sun protection, staying hydrated, and moisturizing can go a long way. Try a facial acupressure massage to relax muscles and relieve tension.

If erasing wrinkles is what you're after, Spiegel suggests meeting with a facial plastic surgeon. "If this is important to you, don't spend your day reading blogs," he says. "Go to a specialist and let them give you an opinion. Ask about the science and find out what works. It doesn't hurt to talk."

There's no foolproof guide to aging gracefully, but knowing what works and what doesn't can help make the process less stressful. If one thing's for sure, it's that worrying does give you wrinkles. However, as noted earlier, don't give up on those exercises just yet. More studies are sure to be coming soon.